Intermittent Fasting

Discover how to Detoxify Your Body, Burn Fat and Lose Weight with the Amazing 16/8 Fasting Method - Weight Loss Strategies to Stop Aging and Live Longer Included!

By

Nancy Johnson

Nancy Johnson

© Copyright 2021 by Nancy Johnson

The following eBook is reproduced below with the goal of providing information that is as accurate and reliable as possible. Regardless, purchasing this eBook can be seen as consent to the fact that both the publisher and the author of this book are in no way experts on the topics discussed within and that any recommendations or suggestions that are made herein are for entertainment purposes only. Professionals should be consulted as needed prior to undertaking any of the action endorsed herein. This declaration is deemed fair and valid by both the American Bar Association and the Committee of Publishers Association and is legally binding throughout the United States. Furthermore, the transmission, duplication, or reproduction of any of the following work including specific information will be considered an illegal act irrespective of if it is done electronically or in print. This extends to creating a secondary or tertiary copy of the work or a recorded copy and is only allowed with the express written consent from the Publisher. All additional rights reserved. The information in the following pages is broadly considered a truthful and accurate account of facts and as such, any inattention, use, or misuse of the information in question by the reader will render any resulting actions solely under their purview. There are no scenarios in which the publisher or the original author of this work can be in any fashion deemed liable for any hardship or damages that may befall them after undertaking information described herein.

Additionally, the information in the following pages is intended only for informational purposes and should thus be thought of as universal. As befitting its nature, it is presented without assurance regarding its prolonged validity or interim quality. Trademarks that are mentioned are done without written consent and can in no way be considered an endorsement from the trademark holder.

Nancy Johnson

Table of Contents

Introduction..8
Chapter 1 - How to Follow an Intermittent Fasting Protocol....10
   Ask yourself why you want to follow an intermittent fasting protocol..10
   Analyze your current eating habits......................................13
   Follow the guidelines for healthy eating..............................15
   Consume more lean protein...17
   Consume whole foods..18
   Include healthy fats..19
   Read the labels..21
   Season your dishes..23
   Avoid popular intermittent fasting protocol........................24
   Avoid certain ingredients depending on your health condition 26
   Move your body..28
   Get some rest..29
   Check your progress...29
   Stop once you've reached your goal....................................31
   Stay positive and get a healthy picture of your body...........32
   Be kind to yourself..33
Chapter 2 - Add more Fibers to Your Intermittent Fasting Protocol..36
   What dietary fibers are..36
   Soluble fibers..37
   Insoluble fibers...37
   Properties and benefits of dietary fibers..............................38
   Importance of soluble dietary fibers: the benefits................40
   Importance of insoluble dietary fiber: the benefits..............41
   Find out how much fiber you need......................................41
   Start with breakfast...42
   Eat the peel of fruits..43

Chapter 3 - Add more Proteins to Your Intermittent Fasting Protocol...46
   Protein powder...49
Chapter 4 - Add more Fruits to Your Intermittent Fasting Protocol...54
   Eat five servings of fruit a day if your intermittent fasting protocol allows for it...55
   Use fruit to snack on...56
Chapter 5 - How to Properly Integrate Vitamin B12 During an Intermittent Fasting Protocol..58
   Eat quality seafood..59
   Do not forget dairy products..60
   Try whole grains..60
   Take a vitamin B12-only supplement..............................61
   Symptoms of vitamin B12 deficiency..............................62
Chapter 6 - How Vitamins Can Improve Your Intermittent Fasting Protocol..66
   Ask a doctor for professional advice...............................66
   Read the label...67
   Take vitamin D supplements..69
   Take calcium supplements...70
   Take magnesium...71
   The role of probiotics..71
   Choline supplements...72
Chapter 7 - The Detoxifying Power of Vitamin C.....................74
Chapter 8 - How to Choose the Right Intermittent Fasting Protocol for You..82
   Low-calorie diet..83
   Low-carb diet..84
   The South Beach diet..86
   Low-fat diet...86
   Vegan and vegetarian diet...87
   Glycemic index diet...89
   Mediterranean diet...90
   Paleo diet..92

Asian diet..93
Diet plans for weight loss..94
Cyclic diet...95
The three-hour diet...96
Avoid crash diets..99
Combine diet and exercise..100
Make sure your diet is flexible and enjoyable....................101
Ask your doctor for advice...102
Conclusion...104

Intermittent Fasting

Nancy Johnson

Introduction

Most women over 50 feel as if they have lost their ability to be attractive, healthy and feel good in their own bodies. But what is the cause for this widespread issue? The fact is that in today's world we are spending more and more time at home and we have significantly reduced our need for food. However, even if we do not need as many calories as we did in the past to survive and be healthy, most of us are still eating as if they were running a marathon a day.

Therefore, it should not come as a surprise that most women over 50 years of age are out of shape, overweight and unhealthy. This normally translates into a worse quality of life and is something that is frustrating for a substantial portion of the female population. Thanks to researches and scientific studies conducted by incredible nutritionists, it is now possible to overcome the negative effect of a sedentary life. In fact, intermittent fasting seems like the perfect solution for all those women that want to burn fat, lose weight and gain a healthy and new lifestyle.

The need of all these women is what inspired the writing of this guide. In fact, in the next chapters you are not going to find complicated explanations of scientific topics that, even if interesting, do not give you a clear direction on what you can do to start feeling better. On the contrary, while writing this book, a great effort was made to make sure that each concept is followed by a subsequent strategy that can be implemented in a healthy intermittent fasting protocol.

By reading this book you will get all the information and practical steps you need to follow to start intermittent fasting in just a few days. We advise you to talk to your doctor before changing your diet as intermittent fasting is not suitable if you have certain healthy conditions.

Please, be aware that the goal of this book is to give you accurate information on intermittent fasting, but it does not take the place of a true medical advice. We hope that you can find motivational and informative insights that help you make a change for the better.

Chapter 1 - How to Follow an Intermittent Fasting Protocol

As we have seen in previous chapters, it can be very frustrating to feel overweight, without considering the associated health risks. You can lose self-confidence and even become a little lazy. To adequately improve health conditions, it is necessary to change diet and choose healthier dishes, controlling the portions. When starting an intermittent fasting protocol, make sure you are getting enough nutrients and avoid restricting your food intake too much. A diet is most effective when accompanied by a healthy lifestyle and the right attitude.

Ask yourself why you want to follow an intermittent fasting protocol

By having all the reasons and goals of your diet clear, you can choose a sensible meal plan that pays off all your efforts.

These are only a few of the different reasons why you might want to start an intermittent fasting protocol.

- Manage diabetes. If you are diagnosed with this disease, you need to change your eating habits. The key to living well with such a disorder is to cut back on sugars or cut them out of your diet.
- Reduce the risk of heart disease. By eating foods that lower cholesterol and help you shed excess abdominal fat, you can decrease the likelihood of heart disease.
- Get rid of the pounds accumulated during pregnancy. It is normal to gain weight when pregnant, but once you have given birth, you can decide to regain your silhouette.
- Get ready for summer. Many women go on a diet at the beginning of summer, when they are terrified of wearing a bathing suit. Sometimes small changes in eating style are enough to avoid this fear and not to be caught unprepared for the costume test.

Before starting any intermittent fasting protocol, you should consult your doctor to be sure that it does not adversely affect your health condition. Tell him that you intend to follow an intermittent fasting protocol. Any meal plan below

1200 calories per day can be dangerous. Michelle May, a weight management specialist, argues that "rapid weight loss from drastically reducing calories results in the loss of fluids, fat and muscle mass. Therefore, metabolism slows down and the body needs fewer calories to survive". In addition, the body tends to accumulate a greater amount of body fat, with the risk of developing metabolic syndrome and type 2 diabetes.

Some women use calories to calculate how much food they should eat, others base their intermittent fasting protocol in grams (of proteins, carbohydrates, etc.), others draw up a list of dishes to eat more often and those to eat less often. Decide how you intend to manage your intermittent fasting protocol.

Make sure your intermittent fasting protocol is compatible with the medications you take. You must be sure that your meal plan complies with nutritional guidelines and that it has no contraindications in relation to the drug therapies you are following.

For example, if you are treating hypertension with the ACE inhibitors used, you need to keep your consumption of bananas, oranges and green leafy vegetables under control. If you have been prescribed tetracyclines, you will probably need to avoid dairy products while taking these drugs.

Analyze your current eating habits

Before starting, you need to be aware of your daily diet. So, try to write down what, when and where you eat to get to know your current eating habits.

Put a diary it in the kitchen or near the bed and write down what you consume (dishes, snacks, small "tastings" from other people's dishes, without leaving anything out), the time and place where you eat (in the kitchen, on the sofa, in bed).

Everyone has their own eating habits and "triggers" that lead them to overeat. Awareness is the first step in learning how to properly manage these aspects when adopting a new meal plan. These are some of the most common triggers for women of your age.

- One of the biggest causes of overeating is stress. When we feel out of sorts or anxious, we often try to console ourselves with food. In these cases, you may want to adopt some stress management techniques or stock

up on healthier foods to keep this trigger under control.
- It is more difficult to make correct food choices when we are tired. If you have a tendency to gorge on food when you feel powerless, you probably want to rest and go to the grocery store once you regain your energy.
- If you have a tendency to empty the refrigerator when you are alone, you may want to consider adding some activity or hobby to your meal plan that will keep you busy outside the home and prevent you from eating compulsively.
- If you skip meals when you have a busy day, you'll arrive hungry at dinner time and eat whatever comes your way. In these circumstances, think about including moments in your new diet when you have the opportunity to eat something in your teeth.

Most dieters find it appropriate to count calories, but another overwhelming majority say they don't actually know their calorie needs. We are used to thinking that fewer calories means losing weight more easily, but in reality it is necessary to be aware of the food sources they come from, not just the quantities to be consumed.

Women report that they consume an average of 1800 calories per day. If you are trying to lose weight, your requirements are likely to be even lower, but you should never go below 1200 calories per day, otherwise the body thinks that it is in a state of starvation, and it begins to store fat.

Ask a dietician or personal trainer to help you figure out how many calories you should be taking in daily to lose the extra pounds in a healthy way. Consider how much physical activity you do during the day. Prioritize foods rich in fiber (whole grains) and protein (lean meats). They will help you feel full for longer and provide you with more energy. Avoid "empty" calories that don't give your body the right fuel. Alcohol and foods such as potato chips are great examples of low-nutrient calorie sources.

Follow the guidelines for healthy eating

The Ministry of Health has developed guidelines in the food sector to help the population to eat properly and follow a balanced diet. In other words, you have the ability to know what the right portions are for each food group without indulging in some of them. In addition, you also need to vary your diet by ranging between different food groups, not just eating apples or other types of fruit, for example. Additional important recommendations include: reducing daily calories from added sugars by 10%; decrease daily calories from saturated fat by 10%; consume less than 2,300 mg of sodium per day. Additionally, there are specific instructions regarding the amount of foods you should try to consume each day, including the following ones.

- Eat nine servings of fruit and vegetables a day. A portion of fruit is equivalent to about 150 grams, which is a medium-sized fruit or 2-3 small ones. As for vegetables, one serving corresponds to 250 grams of raw vegetables or 50 grams of salad.

- Eat six servings of grains a day and make sure half of them are whole grains. One serving of cereal is equivalent to a slice of bread or 80 grams of rice or pasta.

- Eat two or three servings of dairy products a day, but try to choose low-fat ones. 240ml of milk equals one serving.

- Eat two or three servings of protein a day. One serving corresponds to 100 grams of meat, or the size of a palm, an egg, 16 grams of peanut butter, 28 grams of nuts and 50 grams of beans.

- Try the "rainbow diet", which is a diet that varies from the point of view of colors (blueberries, red apples, asparagus, etc.). Each color corresponds to different nutrients and vitamins.

Consume more lean protein

The body needs to strengthen muscles, support immunity and keep metabolism fast. To benefit from protein intake without experiencing the disadvantage of consuming fat, opt for leaner sources. Choose skim milk instead of whole milk and lean ground beef or turkey instead of very marbled cuts. Check for hidden fat in meat dishes.

Avoid whole milk derivatives, offal such as liver, fatty and highly marbled meats, ribs, cold cuts, hot dogs dressed with sauces, bacon, fried or breaded meat and egg yolk.

Let yourself be conquered by the fish. Certain types of fish are rich in omega-3 fatty acids, which are substances that can lower the triglyceride index in the blood. You can increase your omega-3 intake by choosing cold-water fish species, such as salmon, mackerel and herring.

Don't underestimate the beans. Also consider peas and lentils. Generally, legumes are excellent protein sources that do not contain cholesterol and have less fat than meat. Try a soy or bean burger, or add some diced tofu to stir-fried veggies or salad.

Consume whole foods

Whole grains are whole grains made up of three parts: germ, bran and endosperm. Therefore, whole foods contain all three components. Unfortunately, carbohydrate foods undergo a refining process that eliminates the bran and germ, resulting in a loss of about 25% of protein and at least 17 key nutrients. To get all the benefits, opt for foods that are labeled in full on the package.

According to some studies, a diet rich in whole grains has numerous benefits, including reducing the risk of heart attacks, heart disease, type 2 diabetes, inflammation, colorectal cancer, gum infections and asthma. They also help maintain a healthy weight, improve carotid artery health and blood pressure. So, don't hesitate to include about 48 grams of whole grains in your daily diet.

Look for them when you shop. 15-20% of food products on supermarket shelves consist of whole grains. So, look for those that carry the "wholemeal" label or look for a product that is made from whole grains or flours.

Diversify the consumption of carbohydrates. There are not only flour and bread, but also pasta, cereals, biscuits, wraps, scones and other products based on wholemeal flour, so read the packaging carefully.

Include healthy fats

Not all fats are bad for your health. In fact, some should definitely be included in your meal plan. Monounsaturated fatty acids (MUFA) and polyunsaturated fatty acids are appropriate because they provide some benefits, such as lowering bad cholesterol (LDL) and increasing good cholesterol (HDL), but they also help stabilize insulin and blood sugar levels.

Foods high in monounsaturated fatty acids include avocado, canola oil, nuts (almonds, cashews, pecans and macadamias, nut butter), olive oil, olives, and peanut oil.

Eliminate trans fats. They are contained in hydrogenated vegetable oils, so you can spot them if you find "hydrogenated oil" written on the labels. They increase bad cholesterol and lower good cholesterol, with the consequent risk of heart disease, cancer, heart attacks and infertility.

Major sources of trans fat include industrially fried and prepackaged foods, especially baked ones.

Beware of products that pretend to be free of trans fat. For example, in the United States, the Food and Drugs Administration (FDA) authorizes "trans fat free" if a particular food contains up to half a gram per serving. Imagine, then, that if consumption is high, every half gram can become an excessive amount. As far as the European Union is concerned, a regulation has not yet been established that regulates the content of trans fats in food products or the related labeling within the Member States. Trans fats are so bad for your health that New York City has passed a law banning their use in restaurants.

Read the labels

By paying attention to the nutritional tables on the packaging, you can stick to a healthy choice of your foods. One very important part of the table is the portion information: it suggests how many portions are contained in each pack and what the nutritional data are for each of them.

It's convenient, fast and easy to eat out or buy ready-made meals. However, you cannot control the preparation of the food or the ingredients used. One of the most effective ways to lose weight is to cook at home. You can choose healthier cooking methods (such as baking instead of frying) and fresh ingredients.

By drawing up a weekly menu, you will be less likely to let the situation get out of hand and order takeaways in the middle of the week. You can make your life easier by preparing healthy dishes to freeze and consume according to your needs.

Try to enjoy cooking. Give yourself a new set of knives or a cute apron. This way, you will find the right motivation to spend more time in the kitchen.

Don't neglect snacks. Good news! You can indulge in a snack while following your intermittent fasting protocol. By eating more snacks, you can speed up your metabolism and help your body burn more calories throughout the day. In fact, a healthy snack also helps reduce hunger and keep you from overeating at mealtimes.

The secret lies in the choice of food. Consume fresh fruits and vegetables, nuts or low-fat dairy products. Try a few slices of cucumber with chickpea hummus for a satisfying afternoon snack.

Keep healthy snacks on hand when you are at work. If you have some toasted almonds in your desk drawer, you will be less likely to go looking for cookies left behind by a colleague on a break.

Season your dishes

If they are appetizing, you won't be able to resist the temptation to eat them. To add flavor to dishes and stay healthy, try dressing them with some sauce. For example, you could pour tomato puree instead of butter over baked potatoes to lower your fat and calorie intake. Moreover, it is also a way to enrich the meal with other vegetables.

If you season chicken, fish and salads with some sauce, you can make your dishes more varied and interesting. Try buying a fresh salsa at the supermarket or make your own.

You can flavor almost any dish by adding spices and herbs. By the way, they are all calorie-free. Try buying parsley, rosemary, or thyme. They will make your chicken, pork or salad recipes more succulent and original.

In addition to the flavor, some ingredients are also good for your health. For example, garlic has anti-inflammatory properties. Use it to season fish or soups - you'll get a healthy and appetizing meal. Turmeric is another fairly used spice that should never be missing in the pantry. Try adding it to salad dressings to add flavor.

Avoid popular intermittent fasting protocol

It can be very tempting to try the latest trend in intermittent fasting protocols. Often, newspapers and television networks report the experiences of famous women who have successfully tried the most popular slimming treatments. However, it is important to remember that not only are they ineffective, they can also have adverse health effects.

Most popular intermittent fasting protocols focus on one food group, such as carbohydrates. On the contrary, a healthy diet involves the intake of different foods, which is a program that includes the intake of all nutrients. Avoid diets that require you to eliminate the consumption of certain categories of foods.

Some crash diets can harm the body, because they promote a very low calorie intake, causing serious health dangers. Rather, get the recommended amount of calories for your build and make healthy choices.

Avoid industrially produced foods. Processed foods and ready meals are rich in substances that should be avoided like sodium, saturated fats and sugars. This does not mean that a fast food hamburger or frozen food will kill you, but they are foods that you should limit.

The Dietary Guidelines for Americans recommend not consuming more than 10% of calories from saturated fat. If you follow a daily diet of 1500 calories, it means that you can eat 15 grams of saturated fat per day. Fast-food burgers contain between 12 and 16 grams.

Stay away from sugary drinks. Sugary drinks, especially soft drinks, promote weight gain and obesity. The calories that we take safely from the straw are always calories and contribute to accumulating pounds, so try to remove or reduce their consumption.

The most thirst-quenching drink is and always has been water. Also, by consuming more of it, you will feel fuller and can decrease the amount of food you consume during meals. You can improve its taste by adding a few slices of lemon, cucumber, mint or other fresh ingredients.

Fruit juice looks healthy, especially if it is 100% pure, but it contains a lot of sugar. Drink it in moderation or add a little water for beneficial nutritional effects with fewer calories. In a study conducted by researchers at Harvard University, the consumption of sugary drinks is linked to 180,000 deaths worldwide per year, including 25,000 in the United States alone. Another study dating back to 2013, conducted by scientists at Imperial College London, found that the risk of type 2 diabetes increases by 22% for every 340g of sweetened drinks consumed daily.

Avoid certain ingredients depending on your health condition

If you have a digestive disorder that prohibits you from taking certain ingredients, read labels carefully and stock up on products that fit your dietary needs. Follow these guidelines and ask your doctor for medical advice before starting an intermittent fasting protocol.

- Celiac disease. Celiac disease is a chronic inflammation of the small intestine caused by intolerance to gluten, a protein found in wheat, rye and barley. Thanks to a greater awareness of the needs of gluten intolerant subjects, it is possible to find various gluten-free products not only in specialized shops, but also in normal supermarkets.

- Hypertension. It is a dangerous disease that precedes heart disease and heart attack. It can be partly managed with a diet rich in fruits, vegetables and lean proteins. The DASH diet - acronym for "Dietary Approaches to Stop Hypertension", or nutritional approach to reduce hypertension - has been shown to lower blood pressure. It is recommended by various health organizations, including the U.S. National Institutes of Health, and has been ranked the best diet of 2012 by the U.S. News and World Report, a US communications company that publishes news, opinion, consumer advice and market analysis.

- Food allergy. If you suspect you have a food allergy, get allergy tests. Eight foods are responsible for 90% of all food allergies: peanuts, nuts, milk, eggs, cereals, soy, fish and shellfish. If you are allergic, read the packaging carefully to avoid products that can trigger allergic reactions.

While you may be tempted to cut your calorie needs drastically and set high expectations to accelerate weight loss, a slow, determined approach will be more effective and easier to maintain.

Change only one meal a day. Instead of suddenly starting an intermittent fasting protocol, try to introduce only one healthier or smaller meal per day. By gradually changing your diet, you will not feel deprived of anything, but you will have time to adjust to the new situation.

Move your body

A proper intermittent fasting protocol allows you to start adopting a healthier lifestyle. However, you will see better results if you also start exercising. According to some studies, combining diet and physical activity results in health benefits and weight loss.
Try to exercise at least an hour a day. You can break it down into steps of a few minutes to make it more manageable. For example, try walking to work and climbing stairs instead of driving and taking the elevator.

Get some rest

If you don't get enough sleep, you are more likely to gain weight. When you can't rest, your body produces more cortisol, the stress hormone, causing you to seek comfort in food rather than encouraging you to make healthier choices.
Try to sleep for 7-9 hours every night. This way, you will tend to have a healthier body weight than when you only sleep 5-6 hours. Avoid using devices that emit blue light (smartphones, tablets, laptops, and televisions) at least half an hour before bed, as they can keep you awake. Try to keep the pace. If you go to bed at the same time every night and wake up at the same time every morning, you will be more active and rested.

Check your progress

To keep track of your improvements, establish a system that allows you to see how you are doing. The food diary you started writing to keep track of old eating habits can be a great tool to know which way you are headed. Compare your progress, temptations, and successes each week.

Enter all the information relating to your new food plan (starting weight, target weight, daily menus) in a software that monitors your evolution. Many programs also offer healthy recipes and provide forums where you can connect with other people who share your goals.

Check your weight every week. It is not only the daily diet that matters, but also what the scales say. Establish a day a week to weigh yourself and write down the results you have achieved.

Set goals that will allow you to improve your health. To have a healthy lifestyle, you need to learn to set realistic goals. Don't make impossible claims, like "lose 7 lbs in a month". Instead, set smaller, more achievable goals. Typically, to lose weight properly, you need to lose 1lbs per week. Set yourself manageable goals, such as working out six days a week. This way, you will be able to accomplish them more easily and you can reward yourself every time you reach a small milestone. Avoid food-based rewards; give yourself a new tracksuit or a pair of sneakers.

Pay attention to food. Nowadays it is very common to eat while watching TV, checking your cell phone or about to go out, but there is a risk of gulping down more than you need. When it's time for lunch or dinner, eliminate all distractions and sit down at the table. Focus on the food in front of you and appreciate its scent, appearance, taste and texture. Put your fork down between bites to give yourself time to chew thoroughly.

Stop once you've reached your goal

Some intermittent fasting protocols are real lifestyles that can be followed continuously, while others are designed to achieve specific goals in a shorter period of time. Many are fine if they last for a while, but in the long run they risk not being healthy.
Pay attention to the "yo-yo" effect. Also known as weight cyclicality, it is the phenomenon in which the cyclical loss and regain of body weight occurs following various diets. It can cause psychological distress, dissatisfaction and binge eating and, over time, damage the cells that line blood vessels, increasing the risk of heart disease.

Ending an intermittent fasting protocol can be a relief, but if you resume your old eating habits, you risk regaining the weight you lost so hard. Instead, try a maintenance program to stay fit.

If you have followed an intermittent fasting protocol based on liquid foods or which has significantly limited calorie intake, you must be careful to gradually reintroduce solid foods into your diet so as not to traumatize the body. Consume homemade soups, fruits and vegetables for a few days before adjusting to a healthy eating routine.

Stay positive and get a healthy picture of your body.

The strength of positive thinking is not a chimera. In fact, it is crucial to eat a balanced diet. It can keep motivation high, but also energy. On the other hand, negative thoughts can promote bad behavior, such as hitting on food to satisfy emotional hunger and skipping workouts.

Don't be negative. Try not to blame yourself if you go wrong and eat pizza instead of something healthier. Instead, get back on track the next day.

Some days it is difficult to feel comfortable in your own skin. It mostly happens if you are constantly surrounded by extraordinarily thin figures of famous people. However, it is very important for general health and well-being to have a positive body image: it increases your self-esteem and predisposes you to make healthy choices.

Focus on the best aspects of your body. If you love your arms, say it when you look in the mirror. Get in the habit of complimenting yourself at least once a day.

Record a thought-provoking sentence or quote when you mirror yourself. By encouraging yourself every day, over time you will be able to develop a more positive body image.

Be kind to yourself

According to some research, if you are more forgiving of yourself, you will be able to get back into shape more easily. When a negative thought comes to you, try to recognize it and then let it go. It really doesn't make sense to blame yourself for missing a session at the gym. It is much more effective to forgive yourself and move on.

Tell someone (or everyone) that you are following an intermittent fasting protocol. By declaring it, you will prepare yourself to successfully carry out your business, because you will take responsibility in front of others. You may also count on the support of family and friends who will encourage you to achieve your goal.

Stick encouraging phrases on the refrigerator. By having wise words that can lift your mood, you will be able to face the most difficult days of your diet.

Don't deprive yourself of everything that makes you feel good. Go to a beauty center, go to the hairdresser, buy a new perfume. Anything that makes you feel special and pampered can make up for the lack that sometimes creeps in when following an intermittent fasting protocol.

We are sure that if you follow these tips you are going to feel amazing while following your intermittent fasting protocol. At this point you should have all the basic information you need to get started. In the next chapters we are going to dive deeper into specific topics concerning intermittent fasting.

Intermittent Fasting

Chapter 2 - Add more Fibers to Your Intermittent Fasting Protocol

The importance of dietary fiber is considerable. Dietary fiber, in fact, has a series of beneficial effects, such that it is an integral part of any balanced diet in the name of health.

Before discussing in detail the functions of dietary fiber and the reasons why it is important, it is necessary to review what exactly dietary fiber is.

What dietary fibers are

In nutrition, it is called dietary fiber, or simply fiber, all that set of organic substances belonging to the category of carbohydrates (with rare exceptions), which the human digestive system, with its digestive enzymes, is unable to digest. and absorb.

Dietary fibers are found mainly in foods that have a plant origin, such as fruit, vegetables, whole grains and legumes. Depending on whether or not it is soluble in aqueous solution, dietary fiber is distinguished, respectively, in: soluble dietary fiber and insoluble dietary fiber.

Soluble fibers

When it is inside the intestinal lumen, soluble dietary fiber becomes, by virtue of its solubility, a viscous gelatinous substance, with chelating properties against macronutrients such as carbohydrates and lipids. Being viscous, soluble fiber slows intestinal transit, causing a sense of fullness.

The main sources of soluble fiber are: legumes, oats, barley, fresh fruit, broccoli and psyllium seeds.

Insoluble fibers

When found in the intestine, insoluble dietary fiber absorbs water, which has the effect of increasing the volume of stool and making it softer. Thanks to the consequences described above, dietary fiber speeds up intestinal transit, interfering with the absorption of nutrients and reducing the time spent in the intestine of toxic substances for the intestinal mucosa.

The main sources of insoluble fiber are: whole grains, green leafy vegetables, courgettes, flax seeds and dried fruit.

Properties and benefits of dietary fibers

Today, with increasing insistence, experts in the wellness sector, such as dieticians, nutritionists, doctors and personal trainers, are keen to emphasize the leading role that dietary fiber plays in a healthy diet.

In fact, dietary fibers have the following benefits.

- They regularize intestinal function, opposing disorders such as constipation, hemorrhoids and diverticulitis;

- They interfere with the absorption of lipids (fatty acids and cholesterol) and carbohydrates (i.e. sugars), making it a very valuable ally in the fight against obesity and diseases caused by failure to control blood sugar, cholesterol and/or triglyceridemia, such as diabetes mellitus, coronary heart disease, atherosclerosis, high cholesterol and hypertriglyceridemia;

- By speeding up intestinal transit, they reduce the time spent in the intestine of toxic substances for the intestinal mucosa, which has a protective effect against colon and rectal cancer;

- They favor the maintenance of an intestinal pH that depresses the growth of that harmful intestinal bacterial flora, whose activity is a source of metabolites known to be associated with the development of colon and rectal tumors; parallel to this, they stimulate the growth of that beneficial intestinal bacterial flora (prebiotic effect), with protective effects on the intestinal mucosa;

- By causing a feeling of fullness, they increase the sense of satiety, which contributes to better control of body weight and the fight against overweight and obesity.

Importance of soluble dietary fibers: the benefits

Soluble fiber is the type of dietary fiber that is the protagonist of the fight against obesity and diseases caused by the lack of control of glycemia, cholesterolemia and triglyceridemia; therefore, the protective action against excess weight and diseases such as diabetes mellitus, coronary heart disease, atherosclerosis, hypercholesterolemia and hypertriglyceridemia depends on the soluble fiber.

Furthermore, soluble fiber is responsible for that improvement in intestinal pH that depresses the growth of harmful bacteria residing in the intestine, whose activity is associated with colon and rectal cancers, and, at the same time, enhances the development of beneficial bacteria, through a prebiotic effect.

Importance of insoluble dietary fiber: the benefits

Insoluble fiber is the type of dietary fiber protagonist of the opposition to disorders characterized by slow intestinal transit (therefore constipation, hemorrhoids and diverticulitis) and to neoplasms that arise from the excessive permanence of toxic substances in the intestine (i.e. colon and rectum).

Are you getting enough fiber while following an intermittent fasting protocol? Probably not. Do you think that to do this it is necessary to eat only salads? Not at all! Read this chapter to know how to consume fibers while following an intermittent fasting protocol.

Find out how much fiber you need

We have already mentioned the importance of keeping a diary dedicated to what you eat each day, including the amount of food you consume. Research each food on the internet and note the fiber it contains. Here are how many fibers you need depending on your age.

- Men under 50: 38 grams of fiber per day.
- Men over 50: 30 grams of fiber per day.
- Women under 50: 25 grams of fiber per day.
- Women over 50: 21 grams of fiber per day.

If you are currently introducing 10 grams per day, don't jump to 21 the next day. You need to give the natural bacteria in the digestive system time to adjust to your new ingestion. The changes should therefore take place within a few weeks.

Start with breakfast

If it's high in fiber, you can probably add 5-10 grams more to your daily diet.

Eat grains with 5 or more grams of fiber per serving. If you can't stop eating your favorite grains, add a few tablespoons of unprocessed wheat bran or mix them with high-fiber grains. If you like toast in the morning, make it with wholemeal or high-fiber bread. Cook muffins containing whole grains or unprocessed wheat bran.

Add fruits such as berries, raisins, or bananas to the grains to increase fiber intake by 1-2 grams. Swap refined white flour for oat or flax flour if you're making pancakes, and you'll add 1-2 grams of fiber per serving.

If you're making pancakes and waffles, use 2/3 of all-purpose flour and 1/3 of wheat bran. Swap quick-cook oats for traditional oats for an additional 2-4 grams of fiber per serving.

Eat the peel of fruits

Incorporating more fruits and vegetables into your diet will bring more fibers in, but only if you eat the peel as well. For example, don't peel apples or potatoes (in the latter case, use the peels to make snacks). You also need to know that by leaving the peel on the potatoes when cooking them, you will get more vitamins and minerals from the pulp. Do not eat the green parts of the peel, they do not taste very good.

Here are a few interesting meal ideas to increase the fiber intake.

- Dry pea soup, a nutrient-dense food: one cup contains 16.3 grams of protein.
- Vegan roast made with nuts and dried peas.

- Sunflower seed cream and dried peas.
- Iraqi shorbat rumman pomegranate soup.
- Dry pea burgers.
- Spinach and dried peas.

Add whole grains or unprocessed wheat bran to stews, salads, vegetables, and baked foods (meatloaf, bread, muffins, cakes, and cookies). You can also use ground flaxseed or coconut flour, two other great sources of fiber.

Eat more whole grains, which are higher in fiber because the husk was not removed during the preparation process. In addition to providing you with more fiber, they will help you lose weight. A diet rich in whole grains changes your body's response to glucose and insulin, which accelerates the breakdown of fat and makes it easier to dispose of subcutaneous fat, which you can see and grasp.

Replace white bread with wholemeal bread. If you can't, make sandwiches using one slice of white bread and one slice of wholemeal bread. Do you prepare it at home? Replace white flour with whole or half whole wheat flour (use a little more yeast or let the dough rise longer and add an extra teaspoon of baking powder for every 2 cups of whole wheat flour).

Eat wholemeal pasta. If you don't like the taste of it, mix it with the refined one or season it more, but don't overdo it. Eat more brown rice or add barley to white rice for more fiber. You will barely taste the barley, especially if you season rice. Eat more beans, which are high in fiber and protein (which are used to build muscle mass).

Just by following these simple tips you will make sure that you get all the fibers you need to keep your body healthy and in shape.

Chapter 3 - Add more Proteins to Your Intermittent Fasting Protocol

As we have seen at the beginning of the book, protein is an essential nutrient for the development and cell growth of the human body, and is important for supporting the body's immune system. Also, adding protein to your intermittent fasting protocol can improve your health and your overall metabolism, especially if you want to lose weight. The amount of protein you should be getting daily varies based on your gender and health goals. To add protein to your diet, you must first determine the ideal amount of protein to consume each day, and then incorporate foods that are higher in protein into your diet. Use this chapter as a guide to determine the daily amount of protein you need, and find out how you can add it to your diet.

Consult your doctor for the ideal daily protein intake. Your doctor can check the correct dose of protein you should be taking each day based on your health status and the goals you want to achieve.

Eat the right amount of protein each day based on your gender. According to the "Dietary Reference Intake" (DRI) system used by health professionals in the United States and Canada, women over 50 should consume 46 gr. of protein per day.

If your goal is to lose weight, increase your daily protein intake. If you intend to add more protein to your diet specifically in order to lose weight, know that you can take up to 120g. of protein per day; however, this dose may vary based on your gender and health status. Replace the meat included in your diet with lean meats. Examples of lean meats that are high in protein are chicken, turkey, fish, or fillet of meat.

Add cottage cheese to your diet. Each 1 cup (236.58 ml) of fresh cottage cheese contains approximately 28 g. of protein. Add fruit or almonds to cottage cheese to enhance the flavor. Add eggs to your diet. You can choose whether to eat only egg whites or whole eggs; the yolk contains about 6.5 gr. of protein.

Throughout the day, snack on nuts, grains, and seeds. Sunflower seeds, chickpeas, edamame beans, unsalted peanuts, and peanut butter are all examples of high-protein foods.

Add yogurt to your diet. Yogurt is generally a high-protein food, especially Greek yogurt, as it is often denser and richer in protein than regular yogurt.

Eat high-protein vegetables. Examples of particularly high-protein vegetables are broccoli, spinach, cauliflower, asparagus, mushrooms, onions and potatoes.

Eat raw vegetables (such as salad), or cook the vegetables by frying or steaming them. These preparation methods will allow the vegetables to keep all the nutrients and proteins intact; boiling vegetables can reduce the amount of nutrients found in them.

If necessary, use protein powders or protein supplements. Protein powders can be added to certain foods or beverages to increase your daily protein intake, especially if you are having trouble meeting your daily protein intake through the foods you already consume.

Add vanilla-flavored protein powder to your coffee, or mix the powder into foods you cook to enhance the flavor, such as pancakes, oatmeal or muffins.

Since there are many different protein powders out there, in the next few pages we are going to tell you how to choose the best brand for your needs.

Protein powder

One way to integrate protein into your diet is through the use of protein powders. The market is full of protein powders, so it's important to know the differences between the products and choose the one that's right for you.

Before adding protein powders to your intermittent fasting protocol, you should know why you want to do it. This way you can choose the protein or combination of proteins that will give you the desired effect.

Add protein powder to build muscle. They are a great way to help with muscle regeneration and building new muscles. If you are training to gain muscle mass, it is a good idea to add them to your diet. However, a supplement should never replace true food sources of protein. It's all about that, supplements. You will need to use them to add extra protein to your diet that cannot be taken with food.Add protein powder to lose weight. Protein increases the feeling of satiety and fullness, limiting your desire to eat. They are also important for maintaining current muscle mass when exercising.

Add protein powders for your overall health. Studies have shown that some proteins help transport bioactives around the body and lower cholesterol. Adding protein powders to a healthy intermittent fasting protocol can help reduce cholesterol, blood pressure, or fat mass faster than a healthy diet without them.

Add protein powder as a dietary supplement. There are many reasons for adding protein powder as a dietary supplement.
- Vegetarians often do not get adequate amounts of protein and need supplements.
- People who have gastric bypass need extra protein due to reduced nutrient absorption.

- People with certain diseases or disorders, such as celiac disease or Crohn's disease, may need extra protein during breakouts due to reduced absorption by the gut.

Protein is stored in the muscles of the body and must be consumed daily or it will be absorbed by the muscles for biological tissue repair. The result would be the reduction of muscle mass and the loss of strength. For this reason, it is recommended that women take the essential amino acids required by the body every day. Most women living in the Western world don't need extra protein because their intermittent fasting protocol is high in protein. This does not mean that using protein powder is bad for your health, but that you will need to plan your diet carefully, including protein powders as a source of nutrition. Research is still ongoing to determine the exact number of proteins for each of us to consume. However, there are recommendations, based on scientific evidence, that everyone can follow.

Get 15% of your daily calories with protein. Each gram of protein contains 4 calories. So in the case of a 2000 calorie diet, you should eat 75g of protein per day. Again, these are values suitable for sedentary people and the minimum quantities necessary to sustain life. Active people are expected to double that percentage, to 30%.

Increase your daily calorie intake from protein by up to 40% (with fats at 30% and carbohydrates at 30%). Extra protein should replace refined carbohydrates (avoid high fructose corn syrup and processed grains). For a healthy adult, this increase shouldn't adversely affect your kidneys if you drink 12 glasses of water a day. By increasing the calories you ingest with protein, you will receive the heart-beneficial effects brought by these nutrients, burn fat and gain lean mass.

Limit your protein intake to 0.8 - 1.25g per 0.5kg of weight per day if you are looking to gain muscle mass and decrease fat mass. If you have any health problems that can affect your kidneys, limit protein to 0.8 per 0.5kg of weight and consult your doctor for frequent blood tests to check your kidney function. The American Diabetes Association makes this recommendation for people with kidney disease or diabetes. Take note of the proteins you ingest with a food diary.

Intermittent Fasting

Chapter 4 - Add more Fruits to Your Intermittent Fasting Protocol

Eating healthily is a very important part of a healthy intermittent fasting protocol. Fruit is essential to our intermittent fasting protocol because it contains many vitamins, minerals, carbohydrates and fiber. Here are some easy-to-follow tips for getting more fruit into your intermittent fasting protocol and improving your overall well-being.

Eating fruit on a daily basis can help you maintain a healthy weight and reduce the risk of heart disease, stroke, and some forms of cancer. In addition, fruit contains a large variety of vitamins, minerals, carbohydrates and fiber. Hence, eating the right fruit combinations brings significant benefits. For example, an apple contains a lot of fiber but little vitamin C; But if you add an orange and a few strawberries, you'll get all the vitamin C you need for the day.

Eat five servings of fruit a day if your intermittent fasting protocol allows for it

Many countries have adopted national or regional programs to encourage people to eat at least five servings of fruit and vegetables a day. One glass of fruit juice counts as one serving, but drinking five will always count as one serving. If a third of your diet consists of fruits and vegetables, you are well on your way to a healthy diet.

Adding sliced banana to cereal or dehydrated fruit to oatmeal, or making a fresh fruit salad are all great ways to liven up your breakfast. A handful of blueberries and raspberries can be of great benefit. In fact, in addition to the usual benefits offered by fruit, they also contain antioxidants that protect against DNA damage. These include slowing down the skin aging process and preventing sun damage to the skin; a good start to any day.

Use fruit to snack on

Fruit is the perfect food to consume on the go, and can easily replace cookies, cakes and chocolate when snacking. High-fat, high-sugar snacks contain few essential vitamins and minerals, as well as low fiber, and can lead to poor digestion. So, keep some fruit in your car, purse or on your desk at work, to overcome those energy drops that hit you in the mid-morning or mid-afternoon.

Most food manufacturers enthusiastically insist on the fruit content in their food, to make you think it is a great food. Be careful, though. In fact, not everything that has the word "fruit" in its name is what it seems. Remember to check the fat and sugar content in frozen fruit desserts. Canned fruit in fruit juice is usually fine, but beware of canned fruit in syrup, which may be full of sugar. Try to eat five servings of fruit a day for a week. You will see how good it makes you feel.

Eat your favorite fruit within 20 minutes of waking up. During sleep, your body fasts for nearly eight hours. Eating fruit within 20 minutes of waking up rehydrates your body and provides it with low-glycemic carbohydrates that keep your metabolism going throughout the day.

Intermittent Fasting

Chapter 5 - How to Properly Integrate Vitamin B12 During an Intermittent Fasting Protocol

Vitamin B12, also known as cobalamin, is one of the water-soluble B vitamins. Others include folic acid, biotin, niacin, thiamin, riboflavin, vitamin B5 (pantothenic acid), and vitamin B6. All B vitamins play a fundamental role in the production of energy and for this purpose B12 plays an even more important role, which also extends to the production of red blood cells and the proper functioning of the metabolism and the central nervous system. In the next few pages we are going to tell you how to supplement vitamin B12 during an intermittent fasting protocol.

Eat quality seafood

One of the best ways to integrate B12 into your intermittent fasting protocol is to eat seafood. For example, lobster, shellfish and especially clams contain a high amount of vitamin B12. Fish, such as trout, salmon, tuna, and haddock, are also excellent sources of B12. An 85g serving of seafood contains nearly 400% of the daily cobalamin requirement, while an 85g serving of clams far exceeds the daily allowance.

Both meat and offal of beef, such as liver, contain a lot of B12 as well. Pork is also an excellent source of this vitamin. On average, one slice of beef liver contains 2800% of the recommended daily requirement of vitamin B12. Some meat replacement foods such as tofu are fortified with vitamin B12. Consider this option if you are vegetarian or vegan and check the product label for the amount of B12 it contains.
White meats also provide B12, as do eggs. Two cooked eggs contribute greatly to the daily cobalamin requirement.

Do not forget dairy products

To increase your B12 intake, include dairy products such as yogurt, milk and cheese in your intermittent fasting protocol. Some types of plant-based milk are also fortified with this vitamin.

A snack of 250g of low-fat fruit yogurt gives you half your daily B12 requirement.

Try whole grains

Many breakfast cereals are high in vitamin B12. By combining fortified cereals, eggs and milk at the first meal of the day, you will be able to take the recommended daily dose of cobalamin from the moment you wake up.

For example, a bowl (just over 40g) of low-fat muesli with raisins contains 10mcg of vitamin B12, which is 417% of the recommended daily allowance.

Whole grains are a great way for vegans and vegetarians to get B12, since plant-based foods don't contain high levels of this vitamin.

Yeast products and nutritional yeast are excellent sources of vitamin B12. To increase your intake, you can add nutritional yeast to any dish, from cereals to smoothies to evening meals. 5 g of nutritional yeast fortified with vitamin B12 contains more than twice the daily dose of this vitamin.

Take a vitamin B12-only supplement

You can also buy a vitamin B12 supplement in pills. Cobalamin is best absorbed along with other vitamins. Therefore, take it with B6, magnesium, niacin, or riboflavin. In order to get a B12 supplement, you can ask your doctor for a prescription. They may advise you to take this vitamin in the form of an injection or gel.

The recommended daily dose to stay healthy is 2.4 mcg for women over the age of 50. Pregnant and breastfeeding women should take 2.8 mcg.
It is also essential for children, but their needs may be lower than the aforementioned values. The amount needed varies according to age: 9 to 13 years equals 1.8 mcg, 4 to 8 years 1.2 mcg, 1 to 3 years 0.9 mcg, 7 to 12 months 0.5 mcg and from 0 to 6 months at 0.4 mcg.

If you are vegan or vegetarian you should keep the level of this vitamin under strict control. Some women who follow a vegetarian or vegan intermittent fasting protocol may experience a deficiency of vitamin B12, because one of the main sources of vitamin B12 is made up of foods of animal origin. Cobalamin can be obtained through the consumption of fortified cereals. Try eating 3-4 servings a day of B12-enriched foods.

Symptoms of vitamin B12 deficiency

A cobalamin deficiency leads to exhaustion, weakness, diarrhea, constipation, decreased appetite and weight loss. There are also other symptoms produced by B12 deficiency on the nervous system, which include numbness and tingling in the hands and feet, balance problems, confusion, depression, behavioral changes, irritation of the mouth or tongue, and bleeding of the gums. The likelihood of B12 deficiency increases with age, so be careful if you are a woman over 50.

This problem affects women who suffer from atrophic gastritis, pernicious anemia, Crohn's disease, celiac disease, or immune system disorders, such as Graves' disease or lupus. It also occurs in women undergoing partial surgical removal of the stomach and small intestine and in people who drink a lot. Prolonged use of heartburn medications can also cause a vitamin B12 deficiency.

Before taking a vitamin B12 supplement you should talk to your doctor, especially if you are on drug therapy. Taking cobalamin does not involve risks. In fact, in the medical literature there are no toxic or side effects reported. However it could interact with some classes of drugs used in the treatment of gastroesophageal reflux and peptic ulcer. The drugs used to treat these conditions decrease the absorption of vitamin B12. Furthermore, some drugs used to treat diabetes and cholesterol can also reduce its absorption.
If you are taking any of these medications, ask your doctor if you need to increase your B12 intake.

If you have any symptoms of vitamin B12 deficiency, you should see your doctor for a diagnosis. Symptoms of insufficient cobalamin intake can be related to various ailments that need to be diagnosed by your doctor.

If you have been diagnosed with vitamin B12 deficiency, visit your doctor regularly and follow their advice regarding a correct vitamin B12 supplementation.

If you follow these instructions, you will have no issues during your intermittent fasting protocol, even if you are a vegan or vegetarian.

Intermittent Fasting

Chapter 6 - How Vitamins Can Improve Your Intermittent Fasting Protocol

Vitamins and minerals perform several important tasks for the body and are essential for maintaining good health while following an intermittent fasting protocol. Most of the need for these elements is met with food and a balanced diet. In addition to helping you take the recommended daily amount, vitamin and mineral supplements also help you lose weight, but you still need to follow an appropriate and balanced diet plan, as well as exercise regularly.

Ask a doctor for professional advice

Before taking any over-the-counter drugs (or supplements), you must speak to a doctor. In fact, food supplements are not always safe for all people.

Although vitamin, mineral and herbal supplements are subjected to careful checks by the Ministry of Health, they are commercially available without a prescription and anyone can buy any kind. Therefore, it is important to receive the right advice and warnings from the doctor, before starting to take any type of supplement, to avoid unpleasant side effects.

Contact your doctor when you think you want to start vitamin treatment so that you know which one is most appropriate for you. Tell them about the goal you want to achieve with this treatment and ask them if there are other possible solutions besides taking vitamins.

If you want to ask your doctor about the supplements you have already purchased, remember to tell them the brand, the type of vitamin and the format (these are on the package label), as well as the appropriate dosage. This information helps your doctor determine if it is a suitable product for your specific needs.

Read the label

Since there are countless products on the market (not always of certain origin), you need to be aware of what you ingest when taking supplements. Check carefully what you decide to take.

Read the directions for all vitamins. For example, if you are looking for a vitamin D supplement, choose a product that clearly says "vitamin D", then read the label to know all the ingredients, so you know the format and all the ingredients. other excipients present. Make sure other substances are also safe for you.

Check the size of the tablet and the dosage of the active ingredient. Nutritional values should also be included in the label. The recommended posology (for example, 2 tablets) and the amount of active substance contained in each dose (for example, 30 mg) should be indicated. Make sure you know precisely the appropriate dosage for your needs and the correct amount of active ingredients contained in the tablets. Do not take more than the recommended daily amount.

Like prescription drugs, many over-the-counter supplements can also have contraindications. Check for any adverse effects on the label and search online for more information if needed.

Take vitamin D supplements

Studies have shown that people who regularly take this dietary supplement (and were previously deficient in it) while following an intermittent fasting protocol lose more weight than those who do not.

Vitamin D deficiency is a major nutritional deficiency, affecting approximately 500 million women worldwide. The side effects of the deficiency of this important substance are many and include: increased mortality, cancer, metabolic disorders, diseases of the skeletal system, heart problems and infections.

Currently, the recommended daily dosage is 400 IU. However, more recent studies recommend taking up to 2000 IU per day if you are following an intermittent fasting protocol.

Vitamin D is fat-soluble, which means that it accumulates in the adipose layer of the body and can remain in the body for up to 3-6 months. You have to be careful not to take too much, as if it is present in the body in excessive quantities, it becomes toxic and can no longer be eliminated from the body.

Vitamin D is present in few and rare food sources. However, you can find it in the following foods: cod liver oil, fortified milk and orange juice, salmon, beef liver, eggs and swordfish.

Take calcium supplements

Some studies have found that calcium, combined with vitamin D, helps you lose weight. In fact, it has been found that taking large amounts of calcium discourages the accumulation of fat in the cells; in addition, it can bind to some fats in foods, preventing the body from absorbing them.

The recommended daily dosage is 1000-1200 mg. However, you should divide this amount into 500 mg doses, as the body cannot absorb more at a time.

Recent research has found that higher calcium levels can cause heart disease and harden arteries. Pay attention to the total amount you take in through the supplements and foods you eat.

The best food sources are dairy products, dark leafy vegetables, broccoli and almonds.

Take magnesium

It is an important mineral that stimulates over 300 chemical reactions in the body. Studies have shown that, in addition to these functions, it also promotes weight loss.

Magnesium plays an important role in many metabolic functions, but it has been found to improve fasting glucose and insulin levels, thereby helping to regulate weight. A deficiency in this mineral can lead to irritability, muscle weakness and arrhythmia. The recommended daily dosage is 350 mg. Take one or two tablets throughout the day. The best food sources are dairy products, beans, nuts, fish and seafood.

The role of probiotics

Although not considered vitamins or minerals, these are supplements that have been shown to be effective in losing fat and maintaining optimal weight.

Probiotics are "good" bacteria that are alive and present in various points of the gastrointestinal tract. They are ingested through food and drink; their purpose is to strengthen the immune system, as well as prevent or manage constipation and diarrhea.

Several studies have found that consuming various types of "good" bacteria and enriching the intestinal flora are two aspects associated with weight loss and maintaining a "healthier" weight.

If you want to include these supplements in your diet, get ones that contain at least 5 billion CFU (colony forming units) per serving.

You can also eat foods that are rich in it, such as yogurt with active cultures or yogurt to drink, sauerkraut, miso, and tempeh.

Choline supplements

Studies have shown that it helps reduce weight and overall body mass. Choline does not fall into the category of vitamins or minerals, but it is an essential nutrient that acts on metabolism, lipid transport and hormone synthesis.

The recommended daily dosage for a woman over 50 following an intermittent fasting protocol is around 400-500 mg. However, specific choline supplements usually contain about 13% of the active ingredient, but generic ones that contain 3500-4000 mg of phosphatidylcholine (the lead group contains choline) are just as safe.

Among the best food sources of choline are beef liver, eggs, wheat germ, scallops and salmon.

Chapter 7 - The Detoxifying Power of Vitamin C

Vitamin C is one of the most important vitamins for the body; you can get it through your diet by eating foods such as oranges, red peppers, cabbage, broccoli and strawberries. You can also take it in large quantities through powdered supplements to mix with water (or other drinks), as it is believed to be able to relieve ailments such as stress, various diseases and hormonal imbalances. Before you cleanse yourself with this method, however, you need to take precautions and talk to your doctor to evaluate the risks and potential benefits. An abundant intake of vitamin C is not safe for anyone and caution should be taken. However, if you have chosen this option, set up and complete the process within two to three hours; if you experience any complications during cleansing, contact your doctor immediately.

Talk to your doctor if you have irritable bowel syndrome (IBS) or hemochromatosis. If you have IBS or an iron deficiency such as hemochromatosis, you must seek the advice of the doctor before deciding to take a large amount of vitamin C because, if you proceed on your own, these diseases can worsen in the presence of high amounts of acid. ascorbic; your doctor can recommend a specific dosage taking into account your health condition. [1]

You should also avoid this vitamin if you have kidney disease or are concerned that you are allergic to ascorbic acid.

Do not take more than 3000 mg per day. Higher dosages can cause blood clots, kidney stones, digestive problems and other heart-related ailments; you don't have to risk overdosing by taking too much at once. [2]

Doses greater than 2000 mg per day can cause cramps, chest pain, dizziness, diarrhea, fatigue, heartburn and intestinal problems; if you are concerned about these symptoms, consult your doctor before taking vitamin C.

If you are pregnant or breastfeeding, you must be especially careful in consuming this vitamin, as in high doses it can cause hypertension; you must always speak to the gynecologist to find out if it is safe for you, for the baby and not to proceed if you do not have his consent.

Tell your doctor if you have vomiting or diarrhea when you cleanse with vitamin C. If you feel really sick, vomit or have diarrhea when starting treatment, you may be allergic or intolerant to the active ingredient stop taking it immediately and contact your doctor right away. [3]

If you experience a feeling of general discomfort or lightheadedness that does not go away after an hour of starting the process, stop and see your doctor.

Look for buffered vitamin C. Pure powder can be aggressive to the stomach and cause ailments such as heartburn and inflammation. Preferably look for the buffered form, which also contains minerals such as calcium, magnesium and zinc and which is gentler on the digestive system. [4]

You can get it online or in health food stores.

Take powdered ascorbic acid. It is an alternative and contains sodium bicarbonate in addition to the vitamin; this extra ingredient regulates the water intake and facilitates the digestion of vitamin C. [5]

You can look for it online and in health food stores.

Intermittent Fasting

Have plenty of filtered or purified water available. You need it to dissolve the vitamin C powder; you have to drink a lot of it during purification to help the substance travel throughout the body and stimulate defecation. [6]

You must drink at least 5 or 6 glasses of water during the procedure, after which you can drink as many to recover from detox.

Organize yourself not to carry out any demanding activities during the treatment. The whole procedure can generally last from two to six hours, depending on the time it takes for the vitamin to travel throughout the body. Do not schedule outings during this time, as you will need to have easy access to the bathroom to expel the water and vitamin C powder.

Start the treatment immediately in the morning. Proceed as soon as you get up and before breakfast; in this way, the body can absorb the precious vitamin. [8]

Take 1000 mg of vitamin C dissolved in water every hour. Add this dose of vitamin C powder (in buffered form or ascorbic acid) to half a glass of drinking water, mix with a spoon and sip. [9]

If you don't like the flavor of the vitamin powder, you can add some fruit juice with no added sweeteners.

Repeat the treatment until you start producing watery stools. Continue drinking 1000 mg of powdered vitamin C dissolved in half a glass of water every hour; proceed for an hour or two or until you feel the need to go to the bathroom. Check for watery stools this is a sign that you are cleansing your body with this substance. [10]

It takes a few hours for the intestines to start emptying; be patient; you may need to go to the bathroom within 2-4 hours of starting treatment.

Note the times you take the vitamin during the process. Make sure you keep track of the frequency and hourly dosage; that way, you know your vitamin intake for sure and make sure you don't overdo it. [11]

Also take note of when you make liquid stools to better understand how much vitamin you need to detoxify the body, especially if you plan to repeat the treatment in the future.

Consume liquid meals during the procedure. Cleansing leads to better results if you don't eat large amounts of solid foods; opt for fluid foods, such as soups or broths, so as not to create an upset stomach. Continue like this for the 2-4 hours of treatment and gradually return to solid foods when finished. [12]

Drink plenty of water during your cleanse to help the vitamin pass through the digestive tract.

Insert solid foods like rice, quinoa, and cooked vegetables after the "cleanup" is done. After a couple of days, you can switch to more consistency proteins like fish, tofu, beef, and chicken.

Gradually reduce your vitamin intake. Once your body is cleansed, take a smaller dose of the substance daily for 4-5 days; continue in this way until you reach less than 1000 mg / day. [13]

This gradual decrease guarantees the adaptation of the organism to this change and prevents the purification from having negative effects on the intestine.

You may still notice some water in the stool during this phase, but the situation should normalize when you reach a dosage of 1000mg.

Repeat the cleanse every four months or when you start feeling unhealthy. If you have a chronic flu or cold symptoms, follow the treatment every four months or so, sticking to the first-time dosages for best results. [14]

You can also take 50-100 mg of vitamin C regularly to stay healthy; take it first thing in the morning, even before breakfast.

Intermittent Fasting

Chapter 8 - How to Choose the Right Intermittent Fasting Protocol for You

As we have seen, there is a big difference between an intermittent fasting protocol and a diet. In fact, an intermittent fasting protocol is an eating strategy that can be implemented to maximize the weight loss effects of a given diet. However, nowadays there are a lot of different diets and it could be difficult for the average woman to choose the best one for her. In this chapter we are going to examine the most common diets out there to identify which one is the best one for you to implement using an intermittent fasting protocol.

There are dozens of diets in the world, from those that are really smart and in most cases effective, to those that seem to have been invented from scratch and that are useless. In this chapter we will analyze 12 of the most popular diets, ranging from the most restrictive slimming treatments (in terms of calories and food groups), to nutritional styles based on a certain scheme (in which it is necessary to change the times and the way of eating), up to crash diets (useful when you need to quickly lose a lot of pounds). In fact, by having all the necessary information, you can choose the diet that best suits your needs and your intermittent fasting protocol.

Low-calorie diet

It is among the easiest to follow. All you need to do is decrease your calorie intake. In fact, the less you eat, the sooner you lose weight. The assumption behind this eating style is that fewer calories help you lose weight. That said, be careful not to drop below 1200 calories per day.

Advantages. you can eat whatever you want, the important thing is to control the portions. All food packages sold at the supermarket are equipped with a nutritional table. Also, in many restaurants you can find low calorie dishes. In short, it is not difficult to follow it and to integrate it into an intermittent fasting protocol.

Disadvantages. It requires some calculation and some effort, because you will have to keep track of everything you eat and drink, although it should be remembered that technology makes it easier for you. Also, if it is very restrictive, consider that you will not feel full; you may also complain of nausea and dizziness. As if that weren't enough, you'll have a hard time maintaining your weight once you start eating normally again.

Who should follow this diet? If you are determined and have no problem carrying pen and paper with you (or use an app every time you put something under your teeth), this is the diet for you. It is ideal for those women who do not have a large budget and are full of commitments. It is not recommended for those who tend to snack on a lot and for people who hate to constantly monitor everything they eat and drink.

Low-carb diet

It is able to accelerate weight loss, but it is not suitable for everyone. If you follow it, you need to prioritize the consumption of protein and fat (those who support it say that fat is good), so you will eat a lot of meat, cheese, eggs, vegetables, nuts and nothing else. The assumption behind this type of diet is that, when the body has no carbohydrates to burn, it enters a state of ketosis which leads it to directly consume fats (which is why taking them is very important).

Advantages. It is quite easy to follow and allows you to eat many tasty, often fatty foods (such as meat, cheese, etc.), which are prohibited in other diets. There is no calorie restriction, so if it's done right you will rarely feel the pangs of hunger.

Disadvantages. During the initial period (two weeks), people who follow it often feel bad. However, this is a physiological response which passes quickly. Afterwards you feel full of energy, you see an improvement in health and you lose weight. Furthermore, it may be difficult to comply with it because many foods are prohibited. Finally, it can get monotonous, especially if you're not very creative in the kitchen.

Who should follow it? If you know how to cook or are an expert in grilling, you will have no difficulty. It is also ideal for those who do not get bored of always eating the same dishes. However, it is not very suitable for those who love sweets and are not a lover of meat.

The South Beach diet

This diet is similar to the Atkins diet, in fact it eliminates the consumption of saturated fats and certain carbohydrates. Due to its characteristics it is slightly different and some find it more manageable (because the introduction of some carbohydrates is allowed, especially in the second phase).
However, if you are on a low-carb diet, you should take at least 20g per day.

Low-fat diet

In this case, you don't have to eliminate calories and carbohydrates, but fat. It is an eating style that involves some health risks because it excludes essential fatty acids, which are important for the proper functioning of the body. The only fats that are bad for you are trans fats. In short, this diet helps you lose weight because it allows you to take in more calories, proteins and carbohydrates, while restricting the intake of fats.

Advantages. It is quite easy to follow and favors the consumption of fruit and vegetables. Also, in the supermarket you can find numerous low-fat products and avoid those that are notoriously fatty, such as sweets, cakes, cheese, red meat, etc.

Disadvantages. The main disadvantage of this diet is that a low-fat food can contain sugars and salt, substances that are equally harmful to the body, if not even less healthy. Certain lipids are good for your health and there is a risk that the body will want more carbohydrates to fill the gap left by the fat deficit.

Who should follow it? Try it if you like fruits, vegetables, whole grains and lean meats. Discard it if you are a lover of red meats and cheeses, want a meal plan that doesn't involve complications, or are looking for a quick way to lose weight.

Vegan and vegetarian diet

The vegetarian diet prohibits the consumption of meat, while the vegan diet involves the elimination of any product of animal origin (eggs, milk, etc.). That said, there are numerous variations of these two food choices. In fact, there are the flexitarians, who occasionally indulge in meat; the pescetarians, who only include the consumption of fish among their meats; ovo-vegetarians, who admit indirect animal products such as eggs. In general, they are all low-calorie, low-fat, and nutrient-rich diets.

Benefits. This type of diet allows you to lower cholesterol and blood pressure. Most vegetarians and vegans eat a lot of fruits and vegetables, which are ideal for staying healthy. It is not necessary to count calories and sweets are not prohibited. Furthermore, from an ethical point of view they are two diets respectful of animal life.

Disadvantages. You have to be careful. The organism needs proteins that vegetables often do not offer. Being vegan doesn't mean being healthy. Plus, it doesn't necessarily mean you will lose weight (in fact, a vegetarian could technically eat a whole tray of sweets).

Who should follow these diets? Try them if you don't like meat, if you are a good cook (you will have to modify the recipes to meet your dietary needs) and you don't have a tight budget (fresh products can be expensive). Avoid them if you've always been a meat lover and don't want to have complications when cooking or going out to eat.

Glycemic index diet

It is a system that is attentive to foods that can raise blood sugar levels. The higher the potential of a food to raise blood sugar (on a scale of 1 to 100), the less it is considered healthy. A diet like this makes you avoid anything that raises blood sugars, because it is assumed that the glycemic spikes lead to increased fat accumulation, an increase in appetite and weight gain. This diet involves the consumption of complex and whole carbohydrates, as well as some types of fruit and vegetables.

Benefits. It can reduce the risk of diabetes and heart attack. In addition, it favors the consumption of foods that are part of each food group. You can eat as much as you want and when you like as long as the glycemic index is low.

Disadvantages. It is an illogical diet. For example, some types of fruit are fine, while others are not (as if that weren't enough, a ripe banana has a higher glycemic index than an unripe one). As a result, it can be a bit difficult to follow. Also, as the body's reactions to food change from day to day, it can be difficult to monitor its effectiveness.

Who should follow it? Opt for this diet if you are looking for a diet that allows you to lose weight slowly and progressively. Discard it if you want fast results and an easy-to-control diet.

Mediterranean diet

It focuses on the consumption of simple and fresh foods. It is based on the typical diet of Southern Italy and Greece, consisting of numerous varieties of fruit and vegetables, olive oil, non-GMO dairy products, dried fruit and little red meat. Those living in these regions have a lower risk of developing cardiovascular disease, cancer, diabetes and obesity.

Benefits. It does not openly rule out a particular food group, although it leaves little room for industrially processed junk foods. It includes complex carbohydrates, such as oats (great for most people), and occasionally a glass of red wine. It has been shown to be good for overall health and is fairly easy to follow, as long as the follower is aware of the decision made.

Disadvantages. Weight loss is not fast and the effects may be more internal than external. Since it is quite a varied diet, it is easy to assume that a food is fine, when it could be harmful. A handful of nuts is healthy, but a whole jar is not. Sometimes it is difficult to know when to contain portions.

Who should follow it? Try it if you intend to improve your overall health (rather than lose weight quickly) and you like the idea of avoiding processed foods, preferring fresh ones while following an intermittent fasting protocol. Forget if you want a quick loss of weight, don't know how to cook (few frozen foods are compatible with this diet) or have a limited budget.

Paleo diet

It is a recently developed diet that allows you to eat only the foods available in the time of primitive men, namely lean meats, fish, fruit, non-starchy vegetables, nuts and eggs. It totally excludes dairy products, processed foods and starchy vegetables, such as potatoes. It can significantly lower your blood sugar and, therefore, prove to be very healthy.

Benefits. It can promote strong weight loss, as long as it is followed correctly. It is based on the assumption of how humans should eat to get better. Also, don't count calories!

Disadvantages. You cannot eat potatoes and dairy products, because they are included in the list of prohibited foods even if they are generally considered healthy (like milk). Moreover, since some basic ingredients are excluded, it can be really difficult to eat out or have a particular dish prepared. In addition, there is the risk of overdoing it with some dish that is good for you, provided it is consumed in moderation.

Who should follow it? Choose this diet if you are an advocate of healthy eating and like to challenge yourself in the kitchen. Avoid it if you don't have the time and energy to try new cooking techniques or don't want to make a thousand changes to the restaurant menu. Also, it's not ideal for someone who can't live without dessert.

Asian diet

Known as the mother of all modern diets, the traditional Asian diet has a history of nearly 5,000 years and is now practiced by billions of people around the world. It focused on a natural, healthy and balanced diet based on fruit, vegetables and whole grains, with moderate consumption of eggs, lean meat and fish. Those who follow it are also exposed to a lower risk of diabetes, high cholesterol, heart disease and stroke.

Benefits. It is completely natural, based on scientific research and 100% safe. It is balanced to meet all of your nutritional needs. No calculation is needed, but you can do it if you wish.

Disadvantages. You have to learn how to cook some Asian dishes, even if they are generally not complex. You have to give up almost all processed and junk foods.

Who should follow it? It is the perfect diet for those who want to eat healthily and cleanly, learn about other cultures and try new recipes in the kitchen.

Diet plans for weight loss

There is a plethora of diet programs, such as Weight Watchers, Jenny Craig and Nutrisystem, planned with menus, meetings and brochures to help you stay on track and motivated. Typically, they prescribe a low-calorie diet, but some also include low-fat foods.

Advantages. They are tailor-made for you. Some even provide for home delivery of what you need to eat. If you follow them carefully, it will be almost impossible to overshoot. In addition, you can count on a network of people ready to support you.

Disadvantages. In general, you only eat the foods included in the program, which by the way is paid for by the membership.

Who should follow it? Give it a try if you want to have something planned to help keep your life uncomplicated. It is also ideal for those women who need constant stimulation and find meetings and participation in support groups useful. However, if you like to cook and give space to creativity, this is not for you.

Cyclic diet

Recent studies are in favor of this type of diet which is divided as follows. Some days of the week are dedicated to the consumption of low-calorie foods, a couple of days are dedicated to a regular diet and only one to a high-calorie diet. This alternation prevents the body from getting used to the intermittent fasting protocol and therefore the metabolism remains active.

Advantages. There is no exclusion or limitation to any food group and there is a day in which you can "binge in a healthy way". You are not told when you can do it - you just have to organize yourself properly.

Disadvantages. You have to learn how to count calories, which can be a hassle especially in the beginning. You can't even give yourself too much freedom: just because you have a full calorie day, doesn't mean you can eat 30 cookies, otherwise you compromise the results.

Who should follow it? According to most of the research it appears that, when done correctly, it is quite healthy. If you want to see results, just make sure you consume lots of fruits, vegetables, lean meats and whole grains every day, regardless of the day. If you are a committed person and are interested in understanding how the body works, it could be for you. However, you also need to know your weaknesses. In fact, it's easy to give in to temptation, count calories and avoid losing sight of the ultimate goal.

The three-hour diet

You can eat every 3 hours to keep the metabolism active, otherwise the body will automatically run out of reserves. Eat light meals at regular times by adding a few 100-calorie snacks. However, you must avoid eating 3 hours before bedtime. If you want, you can consume precooked foods. As you can see, this goes against a standard intermittent fasting protocol as you can eat every three hours. We thought to include this diet in this list because it could be a viable option for some of you.
Benefits. You can eat everything, including less healthy dishes, as long as you can control the portions. It also helps

you feel full because you eat all day and promotes a good balance between the various food groups.

Disadvantages. It could be easily mistaken. Freedom can lead you to go astray. Furthermore, there is not much scientific evidence to support the effectiveness of mini-meals.

Who should follow it? Try this diet if you feel like trying something different and are in the habit of snacking on a lot. Discard it if you want an effective method to help you lose weight fast or you don't have enough willpower to keep your commitment.

The new Beverly Hills diet
It is based on a very specific idea. In fact, for this diet it doesn't matter what you eat, but what counts is to do it at the right time and make the right food combinations. A correct combination of these two factors promotes digestion which prohibits the body to store fat. Supporters of this dietary regimen believe it is possible to lose 7 lbsin the initial phase which lasts 35 days.

Benefits. Believe it or not, there are no restrictions on calories or food groups. You don't have to calculate your calorie intake, but pay attention to when you eat. In addition to this, the consumption of fruits and vegetables is encouraged, which is good for the body.

Disadvantages. To begin with, there is no scientific evidence to support its effectiveness; in the beginning you can only eat fruit, which is not healthy at all. The rules are a bit confusing and difficult to follow (for example, once you have chosen a protein dish, you can only eat proteins; when you eat a certain type of fruit, then you have to move on to another and so on).

Who should follow it? Try this diet if you don't get along with portion control or food restrictions. If you're willing to splurge, you can buy books, DVDs, and meal plans. Avoid it if you are not committed and diligent.

Avoid crash diets

Crash diets are extreme diets that promise rapid weight loss, but the problem is that they rarely work. They often cause you to starve and, as a result, are bad for your health. When you want to lose weight, try to avoid the following types of diets.

- Purifying diets;
- Juice diets;
- Soup-based diets, such as cabbage or chicken
- Liquid based diets;
- The grapefruit diet.

Regardless of what kind of diet you decide to adopt, co-opt someone else's support if you can. This is especially important if you have chosen a difficult diet to follow. Knowing that you can count on someone is what you need to not lose heart.

This is why programs like Weight Watchers are enjoying some success. However, you don't need to subscribe to a certain program if you want support. In fact, you can just contact friends and family to have some form of support.

Combine diet and exercise

Each diet should be paired with physical activity, whether it's aerobics, weight lifting, or both. Whether you want to walk or run 3 miles, try to get moving. This way, the results will be really visible and it will be easier to continue the diet. Do at least 150 minutes of exercise a week to keep yourself healthy. If you want to lose weight, you should increase the training time to at least 5 hours.

Avoid motor activity only if you crack down on calorie restriction. Exercising continuously on an empty stomach carries health risks.

Whether you are on a diet or not, preferably choose organic and whole foods. The less they are processed, the more the nutrients they contain are preserved. This eating style can be expensive. To save money, buy in bulk or, if you can, shop at a fruit and vegetable store. Also, if you are lucky enough to have friends who are attentive to their nutrition, try to get organized with them to buy larger quantities at a better price.

Make sure your diet is flexible and enjoyable

You will not be able to follow it if it does not have these two characteristics:

- **Flexible**. There will be days when you want to go to a restaurant, days when you have nothing at home but pizza and days when you have no desire to respect your intermittent fasting protocol. A flexible diet that doesn't cause you to feel guilty when you go wrong is easier to implement in an intermittent fasting protocol.

- **Pleasant**. You don't have to be a scientist to understand that it's not the best to drink just water with a squeeze of lemon and maple juice for a week. If it were, it would be a recommended diet for everyone. Whatever type of diet you choose, make sure it allows you to eat foods you enjoy. Do you like meat? Try the Atkins diet. Do you love olive oil? Give the Mediterranean diet a try. The choices are not lacking and your intermittent fasting protocol can be adapted to different diets.

Ask your doctor for advice

The only person who knows your body almost as much as you do and who can give you a reliable opinion is your doctor. Therefore, you need to consult it before you seriously go on a diet. Every woman is different and some diets are not suitable for everyone.

This recommendation is especially true if you are pregnant, experiencing menopause, an elderly person, or if you have health problems. The last thing to hope for is that a new eating style will affect your health in a negative way. So, select a couple of diets that piqued your interest and talk to your doctor about them before implementing them in your intermittent fasting protocol.

Ask your doctor if they can recommend a dietician who will help you make a nutritional plan that fits your lifestyle and weight loss goal.

Conclusion

We would like to thank you for making it to the end of this intermittent fasting guide. We have done our best to ensure that every information contained is useful and helps you in your journey towards a healthier you.

We know how frustrating it could be to start an intermittent fasting protocol and feeling discouraged by the fact that results do not appear immediately. As we repeated throughout this entire guide, the goal of intermittent fasting is to create a healthy lifestyle that can support you over the years, not just give you a rapid weight loss that is unsustainable over the long run.

By following the intermittent fasting protocols and strategies shared in this book, you will certainly burn fat, lose weight and feel much better. However, as we do not know you in person, our final recommendation can only be the following one.

Nancy Johnson

Before starting an intermittent fasting protocol talk to your doctor and find out whether intermittent fasting could be a good idea for you or not. Remember, never sacrifice your health to fit into that new skirt you just got.

Be healthy and your weight will adapt.

To your success!

Nancy Johnson

Lightning Source UK Ltd.
Milton Keynes UK
UKHW041855080421
381687UK00001B/45